MW00898307

Six Simple Steps to Success Vol. 3

Bulletproof Health and Fitness

Your Secret Key to High Achievement

Written and Published By: Michal Stawicki

TABLE OF CONTENT

1. YOUR BODY IS YOUR BASIC ASSET

You are your most precious asset and your body is an integral part of who you are. (You can study the *"You are your most precious asset"* concept a bit further by checking out the free introduction to this series, *Simplify Your Pursuit of Success*.)

Any improvement you can make in the functioning of your body improves your well-being.

You may wonder about my qualifications. I'm neither a personal trainer nor a bodybuilder. I'm neither vegan nor diet specialist. I'm an ordinary guy who takes care of his body among a multitude of duties all of us have: job, family, church, and more.

In my job, I spend four hours a day commuting and eight hours a day sitting behind a desk.

I'm male. I'm 36 years old. Let's check out my body and my health.

I am 5'5" tall (shorter than average). I weigh about 143 lbs. I can do 153 consecutive push-ups or 35 archer's push-ups on one arm. My record is 46 consecutive chin-ups and 43 consecutive pull-ups. I've heard that's quite an extraordinary performance for someone training without weights for only 15 minutes a day. I was last sick in July 2013, with a fever of some kind (plus a nasty case of a runny nose in October 2015). I began taking proper care of my body only about three years ago. I had paid almost no attention to it before.

All of the above indicators point to me having achieved something I call a successful body. The stamina and strength I get from it provides me with loads of energy. I'm able to do much more than merely fight each day for another breath of air.

Among my many obligations, I have a writing career. I began it in April 2013. On top of my full-time job, commuting, family issues, and social obligations, I write at least an hour a day and work on my own personal development for another hour. The most important takeaway is this: I've done this consistently for over two years. Hardening my body has helped me to harden my mind and has freed an untapped source of energy.

Some people don't agree that your body is part of your essence. Referred to as Gnostics, they despise everything in the material world. Among the many crazy philosophies that people have described throughout millennia, this is one of the craziest. Gnostics claim that "spirit" is all that really counts, and therefore, the body is nothing, just pure filth, and anything you do to it is unimportant. In my view, this is lunacy, and I don't argue with lunatics. I avoid them.

Surely, there is nothing more intimate than your own body. Our language clearly shows that we feel this way as a culture. Sayings such things as, *"You get under my skin"* or *"I need to get something off my chest,"* vividly illustrates this level of familiarity.

By changing your body, you can change your whole being, which will have the effect of changing your whole life. This can lead to enormous success. There are a lot of stories out there that illustrate this. Some who successfully transformed their bodies, started new careers or businesses. For example, Isabel De Los Rios, after a fight with obesity, launched her own fitness and nutrition business and is now helping thousands of people.

Transforming your body is sooooo easy compared to the process of transforming your mind. Mastering your body is just a question of a few simple disciplines that you intimately understand: eat less, eat better, move more, drink smarter, and sleep better. It is easy because you receive almost instant feedback after every action. Sleep well at night, and you'll feel better the next day. Start moving more, and after a week or two, you'll notice the things that were difficult—like those dreadful stairs—are easier now. Stop eating junk and you'll notice a difference on the scale after a month.

In contrast, molding your personal philosophy and mindset while painstakingly analyzing yourself is much harder to master because these things are not tangible. You are not used to working actively with your mind, because you spent your life letting your mind do as it pleased. Your mind, on autopilot, has taken care of everything. It filters all sensory inputs and all cognitive impulses (data connected to your beliefs and worldview), and arranges them in accordance with your past experiences and present philosophy.

How close can you get to the time set by the fastest 60 meter runners in the world? How much can you lift compared with the weight the world's strongest person can lift? Me, I'm too short to break the world's weight lifting record. My body is too small and can support too little muscle mass to reach that accomplishment. But a couple of years ago, I had an epiphany. I was participating in the online Transformational Contest organized by *Early to Rise*. Its chief editor, Craig Ballantyne, started his career as a personal trainer many years ago and made a small fortune selling his fitness programs over the Internet. His life has been focused on health and fitness since his university days. During the contest, he announced a challenge: How many pull-ups could any of the participants do within eight minutes? He demonstrated his performance and I beat him by two.

I am a white-collar worker. I spend eight to twelve hours just sitting on my ass behind a desk or on public transport. I was able to do more pull-ups than a man whose job was fitness.

Mind blowing!

Let's return to stretching your imagination. Think of the most lauded physicist in the world. Can you imagine yourself as an equal to this person? I don't think I can. I do have a degree of intellect, so I suppose it's possible that if I put in 20 to 30 years of diligent study I could have similar prowess. Maybe.

But reaching parity with someone who has mastered a specific area of knowledge pales alongside the ability to match the mastery of someone proficient in the realm of soul. Can you imagine yourself exercising the same kind of love as Mother Teresa did? She cared for the sick and the poor not just one time but for her whole life. Could you love everyone equally? When I ponder Mother Teresa and people like her—Nelson Mandela, Mahatma Gandhi, Martin Luther King—I wonder if I am a member of the same species.

It is exponentially harder to master the intangible realm of mind and emotions than to master your body.

I am a bit old school in that I only feel comfortable writing in-depth about solutions that I have experienced myself. Transforming a body is something that I have done well, and the "doing of it" started miracles in my life. For about five years I did push-ups every day. Well, very occasionally I forgot, or was unable to do them because of sickness. That one simple discipline helped me to achieve an amazing transformation several years later.

I started doing push-ups to improve my fitness; I even believed push-ups would help me lose weight. They had no effect on that. But when five years later I read *The Slight Edge* by Jeff Olson, I already had internalized the experience of pursuing a daily discipline for years.

Jeff claims that consistent pursuit of a daily discipline is a foolproof way to succeed in anything. I wanted to succeed in so many realms! But I also felt helpless. I didn't really believe I could improve my finances or spirituality. Those areas seemed to be out of my reach. But my push-ups experience gave me a frame of reference that allowed me to translate Jeff's concepts directly into my life.

If I had not already trained my body for years, I would have dismissed his advice. Not so long ago, the self-help gurus could talk about motivation to me for hours with no effect. The whole subject of mindset and attitude was a foreign concept. I did try many years ago to transform my life using some motivational concepts, but had no success. I had no context; I had no appropriate experience to compare these ideas with.

However, once I had recognized my ability to control my body, I was able to grasp the idea of control over my mind. The almost immediate feedback made me realize I had power over my life. Bodily transformation led to life transformation.

It's hard to come up with anything more tangible, more controllable, and closer to your essence than your body. In fact, you exercise control over your body your whole life. As a baby you learn to use it. As a kid and adolescent you strengthen it and practice your power over it. As an adult you perform daily tasks that form natural paths as deep as the Grand Canyon and strong as the Amazon. It's the ultimate tool that can teach you your power. Of course, it's illusory; even the most powerful man on Earth has a miniscule impact on the universe, but I won't go deep into this philosophical discourse here. Sadly, most of us are taught self-imposed helplessness. Our fears paralyze us. We don't take consistent action to achieve our dreams.

The fast feedback loop that exists between your mind and your body allows you to observe "in fast forward" the laws that govern our society and this world in general. You learn that if you apply consistent focus and attention, you receive results within days or weeks. You learn that *you* govern your body, not the other way around. You become ready to extrapolate this experience into other areas of your life: relationships, career, spirituality, education. There is a greater distance than between your body and you, the feedback loop is longer, so it takes longer to achieve meaningful results or it may require enormous amounts of applied focus to get such results. But the underlying principles are the same: slog and you will achieve, ask and you will be given, seek and you will find.

Taking care of your body is the kindergarten of success; you learn the basics in this "course." The benefits don't end there. Brendon Burchard, now a millionaire, was fascinated by the idea of learning success from others. He was curious about the common traits of successful people. Among several things he discovered was the necessity of taking care of the body's needs. A strong and healthy body produces vibrant energy you can utilize in any way you wish. If you are sick or weak, you just don't have such reservoirs to draw from. Your actions will be feeble. It will take you much longer to achieve the results achieved by folks with high energy. In the end, good health means more time at your disposal. Having a lot of energy means you'll get results faster and will have more time to direct to different projects. And you can certainly save all the time that would be spent on sick leave.

Now that I take good care of my body, I rarely get sick. Except for a slight fever and a runny nose in October 2015, I haven't been sick since July 2013. How many weeks have you spent in bed during that period? You can see the tangible advantage I'm giving myself.

Remember:

- Transforming your body is easy (compared to changing your mind)
- It may start miracles in your life
- Taking care of your body is the kindergarten of success.

2. MODERATION GUARANTEES RESULTS

"Everything in moderation, including moderation."— Oscar Wilde

Quite recently, I stumbled on a silly blog post where a blogger was decrying God for creating everyone alike, when He had infinitive alternatives to choose from. She thought we should have different types and numbers of limbs, and different organs, so we could really accept and respect that everybody is different. But tell me, how could we learn from each other then?

I was fourteen years old when I last attended any biology or physiology lessons. Don't mistake my focus on fitness, diets, or health in general with fanaticism; I am not crazy about these subjects. I'm absolutely comfortable with commonsense knowledge on these issues. Even I know all our bodies are unique. You may be a different gender, weight, and height. Your DNA is surely unique. We have the same hormones in our bodies, but the exact mix of them is unique and affects you differently from others.

On the other hand, it's not as if I'm an alien who knows nothing about your body. Our bodies are alike. We have the same body parts: arms, legs, hands, back, an analogue blood circulation system, a nervous system, and an immunological system.

The specific methodology I used to repair and enhance my body may work for you, but most likely it won't. This is because you are different physically and mentally. My purpose in this book is not to present you with an out-of-the-box "21-Day Program for Rapid Body Transformation." What I *can* do is explain what a successful body is, and which avenues can lead you there. You'll need to be responsible for picking up the pieces that are right for you, the ones that will work for *you*.

There are also personal preferences and cultural differences at play. My thing is HIIT: High-Intensity Interval Training. I'm really reaping the benefits of this regime.

But when I encouraged a friend who wanted to shed some weight to try it, he replied, *"Nah, I hate physical exercises; in fact, the only ones I like are connected somehow with water."* He recognized the need to train his body, but he chose to swim regularly, quite often and long, instead of pushing himself to the limits with HIIT.

When my wife asked me for advice, seeing that I was getting results with weight loss, I advised her to eat raw carrots. She tried it and regretted it. Her stomach rebelled. It worked for me, not for her. Additionally, you may have a different religion, or other beliefs, that will lead you to seek a different diet from the one I chose.

To reiterate: this book is NOT a fitness program. There is no diet you must stick with to get results. That thinking is nonsense. I'll show you the elements I consider important in sustaining your body so your body will maintain *you* in your pursuit for success, and I'll be the first to admit that I don't stick with all of these elements, all the time. I would probably get better results if I did, but I am a prisoner of my beliefs too, even in such mundane activities like taking care of my body.

So, pick the pieces that will work in your case. First, choose those that are immediately applicable. If you cook your own meals, a change of diet is much less troublesome than if your spouse or mum is cooking for you. Next, implement those aspects that are easily adaptable and sustainable. Your body is your lifelong companion; there is not much sense in applying any short-term strategies. Take actions that you will continue doing in the long term. Most importantly, make each strategy your own. Make them part of your constitution, and they will serve you well and long.

If there is a universal piece of advice in this book, it's "everything in moderation, nothing in excess." An excess in anything is rarely sustainable. Your new body will be achieved through building routines, not revolution. As Oscar Wilde suggests, you can overdo even moderation, but in the end, it's the only commonsense strategy when transforming your body.

The ancient Greek philosophers were fond of moderation. Jim Rohn, a man who I admire dearly, who had a similar outlook on health as I have—that it's important, but nothing to be obsessive about—recommended it. My business partner, Matt Stone, who contrary to me is crazy about health and spent thousands of hours studying diets, exercise programs, and a zillion other factors influencing human health, has also concluded that moderation is the best course of action.

Moderation works well for the overwhelming majority.

You're excluded from moderation's omnipotent influence only when your body is special in some way. You've probably heard about people who can eat tons of junk food or sweets without gaining weight. Such people may disregard commonsense dietary advice. You probably can't afford that luxury. In the end, those people would probably benefit from moderation too, as we really are much the same "underneath."

Inevitably, any unusual dietary effect (such as never putting on weight despite overeating) ends at some time, and years of bad habits take their toll. My mum had a "special condition"; she'd never had a toothache in her life. Lucky woman, huh? Well, not exactly. She lost most of her teeth relatively early, in her thirties, because she hadn't been prompted to take care of them. Now she lives with dentures.

A better insight on this moderation issue may be achieved by reversing it: if not moderation, then what? Excess? How is overeating, oversleeping, or overtraining supposed to help you? Then maybe abstinence? What about starving, avoiding any kind of exercise, or continually sleeping only five hours a day? Will such "techniques" give you a successful body?

Bursts of fasting or weight lifting have their place, but they cannot be used as a lifelong strategy.

Remember:

- Choose from this book, advice that is immediately applicable in your situation
- Moderation works well for the overwhelming majority

3. BIGGEST MISTAKE

The most common problem when trying to get your body straight is not a lack of willpower. It's not a lack of motivation. It's not your bad habits or external conditions.

The most common problem is trying too hard at the beginning.

One day, suddenly, you decide to shed some fat or build muscle, and you immediately commence on a crazy regime. You fast for 72 hours, or you go to the gym and lift weights for three hours in a row. If you have ever tried something like this, you know all too well how it's going to end: badly and quickly. After an extended fasting period, or any time on a severely restricted diet, you'll be ravenous. You'll allow yourself too many goodies to compensate. After three hours in the gym, you'll awaken the next morning feeling half-dead, with seemingly every muscle of your body aching.

You may continue this pain-rest cycle for some time, but you won't be able to sustain your crazy regime. And you'll quit.

Yes, quitting is bad … because giving up means you won't get results. In fact it's about the only sure method that *guarantees* you won't get your desired end result.

Why do so many people try this "boom and bust" route anyway? Why are you inclined to lift weights three hours in the gym instead of exercising ten minutes a day, every day? For the same reason that people buy lottery tickets. You want results so quickly that you don't listen to reason. You think that you are "the one in 100" who will actually persist and get where you want to go without a measured, consistent routine.

The overwhelming majority of people would benefit more from putting a couple of dollars into a jar every week, instead of buying lottery tickets. Having a hundred dollars saved certainly beats spending them on thin air. Small and consistent fitness or diet disciplines are better than binge exercising or dieting because they give you the results in the most meaningful time frame—in the long term.

Don't try too hard. I'm sure you have a tender heart; most of us have. But would you leave your whole life right now to tend lepers living in pitiful conditions? I very much doubt you would find yourself able to tend to their rotting bodies and stinking wounds. This is a vocation you need to grow into. Just saying that you care about their fate won't give you the mental strength to pitch yourself into their lifestyle. You must be spiritually and mentally strong to face such a calling. Everything has its own time and the beginning of anything significant is usually done in small incremental steps.

Another mistake many make is thinking fitness is achieved through physical activity alone. Yes, it's your physical body we are considering, but you are not just a heap of proteins randomly assigned together. You are body plus soul plus mind. Viktor Frankl[i], a world-class psychiatrist, claimed that if you focus solely on the physical side of things, you are bound to be surprised by a sneaky attack from your mind. You can have the perfect exercise routine planned for months ahead, but then some unpleasant event will take place and your mind will betray you. It will talk you out of exercises and talk you into an ice-cream treat, because "you deserve it."

Mind games alone won't work either, of course. You'll achieve little by murmuring mantras such as *"my body is in vibrant health and leads me to success"* or *"my muscles are getting stronger with each thought I feed them."* You need to plan and execute your diet, exercises, sleeping schedule, and so on.

Mindset is important, but it's only a piece of the puzzle. Don't neglect the doing.

You may wonder what kind of attitude is best when trying to transform your body.

The answer: one that welcomes consistency and is focused on the long term. Your body will be with you to the end of your days. You eat, sleep, move, and drink every day. You must develop appropriate habits regarding those activities; otherwise, you'll be in for a lifelong struggle, or for failure. Losing 40 pounds this year, or being able to bench-press 200 pounds in six months, will not change the grand scheme of things if you don't design a support system for such achievements. Next year you might gain 50 pounds. Rapid results are great. They boost your self-confidence and, if your body is shape, such results awesomely energize you. Sustainability, should be your main concern.

Getting a long-term mindset is relatively easy if you can observe the results immediately (in human life-expectancy terms). When I decided to start my indie author career, I had a raw draft of my first book finished within a month. It took me six weeks to publish it, and ten weeks to get some meaningful data about sales. Based on that data alone, I would have to conclude it would be about 30 years before I could sustain myself financially by writing.

However, when I replaced sweets with raw carrots, I saw a scale moving downward within a month. One month is statistically only about 0.02 percent of your life. It's hard to imagine any other area that rewards activity with such clear, rapid feedback.

Your body is so close to you and you have so much influence on it, that it's an order of magnitude easier to observe and reap the benefits of perseverance. Working to improve your body will teach you the benefits of consistency within weeks.

Remember:

- • The most common mistake is trying too hard at the beginning
- • Fitness is not achieved through physical activity alone (neither through pure mental activity)
- • Consistency and focus on the long term is a winning attitude when it comes to taking care of your body.

** FREE BONUS **

To download a single PDF sheet describing how I avoided the biggest mistake, visit:

www.ExpandBeyondYourself/mistake

4. YOUR LIFE IS MADE OF HABITS

The word **habit** comes from Old French *abit*, *habit*, from Latin *habitus* "condition, appearance," from *habere* "have, consist of." The term originally meant "dress, attire" and the noun habit meant a monk's outfit. The habit was an external sign of a monk's internal constitution that defined his whole life. Later, the meaning of this word drifted, and now also means physical or mental constitution.

In other words, habits are part of your being. Habitual activities are those that are ingrained in your core being and, in the end, they define who you are. When you understand this, you'll know you can remodel yourself by rebuilding your habits. Develop any new good habit and your own constitution changes. You will become someone slightly different. Repeat this process one habit at a time and you will become a different person. You may be horrified by the thought of intervening into your internal constitution. But you shouldn't be. We are not a static species; we constantly adjust to the external world.

By taking control over your habits, you just take conscious charge of this process.

There are two mainstream schools when it comes to building new habits.

1. Tiny habits.

This term was invented by BJ Fogg from Stanford University. He defines tiny habits as activities that

- you do at least once a day,

- take you less than 30 seconds,

- require little effort.

Behind his methodology stands a whole philosophy of habit forming, common to many personal development advisors, from Fogg's "competitor," Stephen Guise, who popularized the concept of mini habits, to Charles Duhigg, the author of *The Power of Habit*, to Leo Babauta. This school of thought encourages you to carefully design your new habits based on the science of human behavior, focused on consistency and habit development itself rather than immediate results. It recommends starting small and, in increments, building your habits gradually.

I'm a firm supporter of any method that helps develop consistency, because I believe it is a core success trait. There is a lot of merit in that approach. Connecting habits to results is not reasonable because you'll expect results too soon in most cases. Well, perhaps your conscious mind will not be expecting them, as you know your first workout won't give you a model's body. But try to explain it to your monkey brain. The conversation will go like this:

Stage A, before the workout:

"Workout! Workout! Wonderful! I'll no longer be a fat ass! I'll become the Hulk! Yippee!"

Stage B, during the workout:

"Heck, this is no fun! I hurt! I'm short of breath! I'll suffocate! I should stop right now!"

Stage C, immediately afterward, in front of a mirror:

"WTF? My fat is not gone! And it was so much effort! It was so much pain! Oh, no, no! I won't support this stupid plan anymore!"

When you focus on consistency, the results will come. And you will explain to your monkey brain that you aren't pursuing the body of Hulk, but simply want to get the next workout done. Then it will be satisfied:

"Well done! I've done another workout, exactly to the plan! I'm very successful! Another accomplishment under my belt!"

What is more, tiny habits won't make your monkey brain scream in pain. Tiny habits are ideally suited for the mind's reward system. You will draw satisfaction from fulfilling your small disciplines. Tiny effort and a lot of joy, that's something your monkey brain definitely understands. After an initial period, your subconscious will adopt the new habit as a part of your identity because it will be your source of positive feelings.

2. Maxi habits.

That's my name for what we usually try to accomplish when starting new habits.

Consider your own experience. At the beginning you are usually ambitious. You want to start strong and get rapid results. You decide to starve yourself for a month or go to the gym every other day. The advantages of this approach are obvious; that's why so many pursue it. It seems natural: if you sow a lot, you will reap even more. After last Christmas I fasted 96 hours straight. I didn't allow even a single crumb into my body. I lost about 7 pounds. That's a maxi approach at work.

The same may be done in the case of exercise. After a month of weight lifting, you will surely notice some change in your body image. However, your muscles are much less inclined to cooperate and grow at a rapid pace. The problem with this approach is that it's not sustainable. You can't exercise a few hours every other day; you have a life to live.

You surely don't intend to spend your life in a gym. And you can't fast forever. You have to eat something.

Once you go off any rigid discipline, you are much more inclined to compensate yourself for the struggle you went through. The yo-yo effect seen in dieting is a perfect example of such behavior. It's normal. And it's dangerous.

You'll see the yo-yo if you're doing this two-step dance: First, you fast rigidly for a few days or diet for a few weeks, mobilizing your willpower and experiencing pain. Then you stop, and overcompensate. After another few days or weeks of binge eating, your weight is back at its prior level. The yo-yo can be discouraging and off-putting. What was your struggle for if you are back where you were?

The negative effect doesn't just stop with one zero net result, either. You'll begin thinking that habits, in general, suck; or that maybe you are not good enough.

Maxi habits are activities defined as ones that

-need mobilization of a great amount of your willpower to start at every repetition,

-take long stretches of time,

-provide (relatively) rapid results,

-are sustainable only through continuous investment of time and willpower.

Both kinds of habits have their place. Maxi habits are necessary when pursuing a career. Careers are a vital part of life, so they naturally receive a lot of attention and resources.

In case of a health or body-related career, such as bodybuilding or personal training, I'm sure you'd need to commit long hours to train your body and be pedantic about what you eat. A person pursuing such a career must develop the relevant maxi habits, like exercising a couple hours a day, to be successful.

The same goes with any other career. My present day job is database administration. Every time I have a non-standard task, I need to learn something new, usually by searching Google. So I have a habit of researching and learning about 30 minutes a day. Someone who works as a manual worker in a factory may think this effort unnecessary; in my kind of job, it's a must.

Tiny habits are better suited for developing new habits that are additions to your current lifestyle. If you are not a professional basketball player, spending ten hours a week practicing free-throws is definitely overkill. But maybe you enjoy a weekly game with your friends and would like to get better at this particular element of basketball. So each time you get home from work, you shoot a few free throws to the basket near your garage.

3. Ten-minute habits.

I think there is a middle path.

Ten-minute habits, or "midi habits," combine advantages (and dangers) of both above approaches. I give just ten minutes to a single habit every day. It's a relatively short period of time, so my mind is less likely to rebel.

You can do this; you can easily squeeze a ten-minute chunk of time into your schedule. The results are not dazzling, but they are bigger than tiny.

One of the first ten-minute habits I adopted was a speed-reading practice. Within a month, my reading speed increased about 50 percent. Committed speed-readers might consider my progress laughable and slow, but it took very little of my time. As I write this, I'm still keeping up a ten-minute practice session each day. I've probably progressed as far as I can with such a small time investment. But I'm about 100 percent better than I was prior to my daily practices. And I've read about a couple dozen books during my practice sessions I wouldn't have read otherwise.

Ten minutes is just a rule of thumb. You may construct your habits in different units; you might choose two or sixteen minutes. What makes them midi habits is that they are between the two extremes of very small or very large habits. They utilize tiny habit flexibility and minimal mind resistance, while providing exponentially bigger results than tiny habits. But your commitment is larger than required with a tiny habit, so your subconscious resistance may be much higher. Naturally, with less time input, your results will be slower to come. You may be more at risk of short-term discouragement, increasing the likelihood you'll quit. However, combing elements of mini and maxi habits can help you adopt a new habit easier and get meaningful results faster.

I advise this approach if you are impatient, but you tend to start things too ambitiously and give up quickly. I also recommend it in the areas that are of a vital importance for you. I cultivate just five such habits on a daily basis.

A couple of them address my spiritual life: I study the Bible and read from a book written by a saint every day. Both these activities are not only important for me, but enjoyable too. I just love to read and learn.

I also repeat my personal mission statement every day. There is nothing of more importance than my mission.

I practice speed reading (I love reading).

I exercise about five to fifteen minutes a day.

Yes, I've tried instituting other habits. I started and abandoned a few other midi habits; I stopped because none were very important to me. For example, I was studying professional documentation for my day job, but since I've decided to pursue writing as my full-time work, becoming proficient in my day job is no longer a priority.

Remember:

- • Habitual activities are those that are ingrained in your core being and, in the end, they define who you are
- • Tiny habits don't need much willpower or energy, but they also don't provide impressive results; they are focused on consistency
- • Maxi habits are sustainable only through continuous investment of time and willpower; they are reserved for the vital areas of your life, like pursuing a career; they provide relatively rapid results
- • Properly designed ten-minute habits can maximize advantages of both above approaches and decrease dangers related to them.

** FREE BONUS **

To download a single PDF sheet describing how I develop my 'healthy' habits, visit:

www.ExpandBeyondYourself/habits

5. SLEEP QUANTITY

The quantity of your sleep is utterly important. We notoriously under-sleep. If you are anything like the average American, you sleep about seven hours. One century ago, this number was nine hours. There are studies that estimate that sleep deprivation costs the US economy over $200 billion. People who don't get enough sleep are not productive. Other research, by University of Pennsylvania and Washington State University, concluded that if you sleep six hours a day for two weeks your performance is equal to that of a person who hasn't slept for 48 hours. What is more, you are not able to realize your poor performance in that case! The sleep deprivation sneaks up gradually and you don't notice how sluggish you've became.

I don't sleep enough. This chapter is definitely an example of *"do as I say, not as I do."* I try to get at least seven uninterrupted hours of sleep a night, but with my day job and long commute, it's next to impossible. I sleep as little as four hours sometimes, and I'm happy if I get six and a half hours of sleep a night during the workweek.

How long should you and I sleep? Collected wisdom suggests the answer is about eight hours a day. Sleep needs are individual, but they are also predictable for the majority of the population, who don't suffer any extreme conditions or are not gifted with a special kind of mind and body that don't need much sleep.

To get motivated to extend your time in bed, first you must realize how important sleep is for optimal functioning. I hope the results of the research I've referenced have made this clear. Once you know you need more sleep and you've taken a decision to sleep more, you can take care of technicalities.

Surprise, surprise, to sleep longer you need to go to bed earlier. How can you achieve this? There are numerous methods, but most of them come down to the evening ritual. You are a creature of habit. The average urban dweller has a mess for an evening ritual. One night you'll watch TV for too long; on another you'll work till late. In the middle of the week you'll go out with friends or your spouse to eat, returning late. And Friday nights are a whole different story. With no structure or routine, you get random sleep patterns. And you probably don't sleep long enough during the week so you lay in the bed till noon on Sunday.

If you have a structured life, it will be easier to improve things. When you work the same hours every day, a proper evening routine is just an extension of your day. It's more complicated when your working day varies significantly. For years, I've worked on shifts; a three-hour variation between starting at 7 a.m. or 10 a.m. makes more than a minor difference in my daily routine. To add insult to the injury, my kind of work demands working late in the night at least once a month, and sometimes I'm required to work the entire night.

Tough luck.

If you are self-employed and have power over your schedule, it's a bit easier to develop a standard evening routine.

No matter if your life and schedule are chaotic or orderly, a new routine won't appear all by itself. You need a conscious decision and some effort to make it happen. It has to be a design, not a whim. Turning off all your electronic devices in the evening helps your body to quiet down. Did you know that you have photosensitive cells in your skin that allow your body to determine what time of day (or night) it is? Avoid exposing yourself to artificial sources of light like TV or computer screens at least half an hour before you go to sleep. Stay away from sensory inputs, such as engaging entertainment, that stimulate your mind, which cannot quickly be put to rest after.

I spend half my life in front of a computer, but in the hour before going to sleep, I use my computer just to mark off my habits in the Coach.me application. I don't read emails; I don't browse on Facebook or Twitter; I don't read or work (unless I have to).

My evening ritual consists of a few activities, not necessarily performed in the same order. I write in my gratitude journals, I bathe, I brush my teeth, I pray with my kids, I close the door to our house, I mark off habits in Coach.me, and I turn off the computer. I keep my laptop away from our bedroom; it stays downstairs in my home office. The last thing I do before going to sleep is pray. I pray during the evening physical activities like brushing teeth too. I finish my prayer lying in bed. While not intending to, I often fall asleep before I finish my prayers.

Needless to say, part of my "evening" routine is avoiding caffeine after 2 p.m. Its effects can last as long as eight hours.

As you can see, there is a very small space for technology in my evening routine. I also focus on the bright side of life in the last half hour of my day. Gratitude journaling and prayer soothe my mind. When I get to bed, I am already relaxed.

Remember:

- The quantity of your sleep is utterly important
- You need about eight hours of sleep a day on average
- To sleep longer you need to go to bed earlier.

Action Items:

- Design your own evening ritual.

** FREE BONUS **

To download a single PDF sheet describing how I take care about my sleep quantity, visit:

www.ExpandBeyondYourself/quantity

6. SLEEP QUALITY

Your quantity of sleep is the most important. Quality is a secondary consideration. It doesn't matter if you sleep like a baby if you sleep only five hours. Quality can replace quantity only to a certain degree. Strangely, the opposite is true. Get enough sleep, and you need not worry about its quality.

I have to admit that I'm far from an expert in the field of sleep quality. I sleep like a baby, so I don't need to know all this stuff. I have more interesting and urgent areas to study. I find expert knowledge about sleep quality to be highly confusing. Google the phrase and you will get a mishmash of contradicting data. In the last few months I've read in one source that sleep cycles are two and a half hours long, while in other sources I read that they are one and a half hours long. It seems that even scientists can't agree on much these days.

The same chaos rules on the subjects of fitness and diet advice.

Therefore, I invite you to do what any reasonable person should do when met with contradictory advice: filter my suggestions through your experience, try my ideas one by one, and continue implementing the things that work. After all, we are talking about your body and your routine, not about the behavior of laboratory rats!

I think you'll find intuitive knowledge more useful than anything purely theoretical.

So, what do you need to sleep well? In my view, three things: darkness, silence, and peace of mind. Difficult though it may be to achieve, try to have all those factors in play together.

1. Darkness

Darkness is relatively easy to achieve. You need it because you have light receptors in your skin. It's not enough to use an eye patch. If your skin is exposed to sunlight while you sleep, those receptors will send to your mind a signal that the sun is up and it's time to go out from the cave.

2. Silence

Silence is quite obvious, isn't it? It's hard to fall asleep in a noisy environment. Well, you can train yourself to get some sleep when you are used to the specific background noise. That's how people are able to function while living near train tracks. I can sleep in almost every public transportation vehicle. The combination of a vehicle's motion rocking my body and the background music I use to cut myself off from the chatter of co-passengers is my secret weapon. When I also add the mantra of my personal mission statement to the mix, I fall sleep within minutes. However, I wouldn't call those commute naps a quality sleep. They have a place in my sleep routine, but they can't substitute for a full night's deep sleep.

Sound is important for your sleep because it's the last of your senses to deactivate when you go to sleep and the first one to activate when you wake up. Scientists speculate that hearing was necessary in prehistoric times because it allowed people to be alert to danger while sleeping. I see additional advantages: it's also handy for hearing that your baby has woken up and is hungry.

If you want to sleep well, secure yourself a silent environment. Make your bedroom an island of silence.

3. Peace of Mind

The last but most important factor is peace of mind. If you are stressed, excited, or stimulated by events, it's hard to fall asleep. Neither silence nor darkness will help much in such cases. You must calm down before you go to bed. The methods I briefly mentioned in the previous chapter—prayer, visualization, gratitude, dreams, and meditation—can all contribute to ease burdens from your shoulders. Sleep is not merely for resting your body, it's for resting your mind. Thinking about your problems in bed is like trying to get physical rest by weight lifting.

I know that the advice "stop worrying" is easier said than done. Fortunately, you can use an interesting mind trait to help you. You can't think about two things at the same time; minds only have one active track. What is more, you have power over your thoughts; you can force a train of your thoughts into any desired direction. The activities given in the previous paragraph are the tools to steer your thoughts away from problems, stress, and fears, in the direction of hope, joy, and peace.

Prayer.

I recommend it. However, this book isn't a prayer workbook.

Visualization.

You can use it both to dream about the better future or just to imagine yourself in a peaceful environment of your choice, like a seaside or forest in the summer. Keep the image you've visualized in your mind for a few minutes while breathing deeply.

Gratitude.

The easiest and fastest method to practice gratitude is a gratitude journal.

Your "journal" doesn't even have to be a real journal. When I started practicing gratitude, I just wrote a few entries on sticky notes. Sit down with pen and paper and think for a minute about the things you are grateful for, today. When you start this, you may face challenges identifying things you're grateful for. We usually occupy our minds all day long with long lists of things we are afraid of or worried about. If you can't figure out a reason for feeling grateful, then may I suggest you just write down that you are glad this day is over.

However, I believe everything is a possible source of gratitude: your health, family, job, relationships, environment, food, games, shelter, mind, accomplishments, emotions. If you train your mind to find positives, I'm sure you will find, in time, a stream of gratitude coming from your thoughts.

Of course you are not restricted to the journal in expressing your gratitude. You don't even have to write down your reasons for being grateful, but I do think noting them down is superior than just keeping them in your mind. You solidify those reasons in your memory when you write them down. And if you write these thoughts down, you can refer back to them when you have especially bad days.

Dreams.

You can give your dreams a physical presence with a vision board, or a vision journal. Anything that shifts your focus from your present shortcomings and gives you some hope is helpful. If you don't dream about a better life, nobody will dream it for you.

Meditation.

The whole goal of meditation is to calm your mind, to take control of it. Practicing meditation will also provide you with a greater control over your thoughts, not just during those few minutes, but throughout your day. Over time, a practice of meditation makes it easier for you to govern your mind.

What you shouldn't do is to indulge yourself with pleasures to "forget about your worries." Alcohol, drugs, sleep pills, video games, and TV won't make your worries disappear. Those worries will just move into the background temporarily. They will be back sooner rather than later and then they will be accompanied by the unpleasant consequences you've brought on by giving in to your "pleasures." What is more, the human constitution demands more stimulation with time. When you depend on external sources of mollification, you can never get real peace, as that comes from within. If you are reliant on external input, you are in trouble.

To get a good quality sleep, focus on those three factors. Try to improve the soundproofing qualities of your bedroom. Sometimes a simple thing like a rubber seal for the door or windows can make a huge difference. Avoid exposing yourself to electronic lights before going to bed. Consider banning electronic devices from your bedroom. Try to secure a pitch-black environment for sleep. Invest in dark curtains or high quality roller blinds. And most importantly—calm down.

Remember:

- The three factors contributing toward sleep quality are darkness, silence, and peace of mind
- Stop worrying
- Don't indulge yourself with pleasures to forget about your worries
- Consider banning electronic devices from your bedroom.

Action Items:

- Incorporate at least one of the relaxation techniques into your evening routine: prayer, visualization, gratitude, dreams, meditation (or develop your own)
- Brainstorm methods to calm down before sleep; implement one ASAP.

7. HACK FOR UNDER-SLEEPING

Life has an uncanny ability to get in the way. What then? Should you resign from keeping your body in the optimal state? Not at all.

You need to nap from time to time, especially if your life is not very structured. Yesterday I woke up 5:05 a.m., relatively late for me, because the day before, my wife had hosted a small party with her cousin and friend. I slept only about six hours that night. I was on "entertaining duty," so my usual daily schedule went to hell.

I'm lucky that in my office an occasional nap behind the desk brings only sarcastic remarks rather than reprimands. I lost my consciousness for about fifteen minutes in the morning and I was able to work intensively the rest of the time. But when I finally got at home at about 6 p.m., I took a 25-minute nap. I intended to nap a bit longer, but my kids and wife were noisy. Then I worked from 10 p.m. to 3 a.m. I took three naps during that time when the big database files were copying. Today I've slept only 5.5 consecutive hours. It's Saturday, so I did my working routine and sat to write my daily quota of 1000 words. I'm sure I will make use of another nap or two to survive this day. I plan to sleep seven to eight hours tomorrow, on Sunday.

Lots of successful people use short breaks during the day to take a nap and invigorate themselves. John D. Rockefeller and Winston Churchill were well known for this habit. Rockefeller built his empire from scratch and became the richest man in the world in his time. Churchill took naps when he was a prime minister, while governing a nation involved in a war of survival. Those men understood that their bodies are not machines, that they need a break, that their performance suffers if they forcefully stay awake.

You can of course try to use stimulants, like coffee, and sometimes they are useful. You can't take a nap in lieu of an important meeting with your CEO. But as with agents of indulgence and peace of mind, if you regularly use stimulants, you'll need them more and more. A nap is the natural way to reenergize you. After a big coffee I'm animated for about a couple of hours and then the fatigue comes back. After I took my 15-minute nap behind the desk, I am functioning, fully alert, from 10 a.m. to 6 p.m.

As with everything else, scientists can't agree on anything about naps. They can't even determine if naps are harmful or supportive. I've read serious research that concluded that naps are downright damaging to your body. Then there is the question of the nap's duration. Some says that 5-minute naps are OK, others that you should nap at least 20 minutes. What is interesting is the agreement by most researchers that sleeping over 30 minutes at a time beats the nap's purpose, because it actually decreases your performance.

This is all bollocks, in my view.

The main argument against longer naps in these studies is that naps don't increase performance and might even decrease it; that after an extended nap people feel groggy and they feel more inclined to sleep even longer, than to work. I have no idea about their methodology, but I'm far from convinced about their results. Yes, it sometimes happens that I feel sluggish after a longer nap. But this feeling is gone within five minutes of waking up and moving my ass. I have a lot more energy afterwards than before I took the nap.

I don't have time to consider and reflect on every sleep researcher's conclusion. When I feel exhausted and have at least five minutes available, I nap. If I only get five hours of sleep in the night (which is happening all too often) and I can take a 50-minute nap after coming back to home or on a train from work—I just do it.

I appreciate theorizing, but when it comes to my napping, I have only one rule: I nap as long as I can. Yes, I prefer to sleep seven and a half hours in the night and avoid the necessity of naps. Yes, I understand that too much napping, like too much of everything, can be harmful. But most of the time I just have no choice, no power over my schedule, like with this night work I performed yesterday. I work eight hours a day and commute four more, and I have a life outside of my job. Family. Church community. A home to take care of. Appointments.

I sleep whenever and wherever I can, and I recommend the same approach to you.

Your biggest takeaway from this chapter should be this: nap as often and as long as you need and can; ignore research that doesn't match your real-life experience.

Remember:

- Lots of successful people use short breaks during the day to take a nap and invigorate themselves
- Most research agree on 5–25 minutes being an optimal nap's length.

Action Items:

- Lots of successful people use short breaks during the day to take a nap and invigorate themselves
- Most research agree on 5–25 minutes being an optimal nap's length.

** FREE BONUS **

To download a single PDF sheet describing my napping strategy, visit:

www.ExpandBeyondYourself/naps

8. DIETS DON'T WORK

Let's talk about food. Am I a diet or nutrition expert? No. Should I be to be able to provide some commonsense advice? Yes.

We are crazy about "certified" this or that, but all of us eat! This is one of the most basic human needs. Every day billions of people consume millions of tons of food without being certified in nutrition.

My experience with food won't give you the tips you need to become a super-thin fashion model or the top world's athlete. However, I've discovered a few things that have helped me maintain a high energy equilibrium, and I think you can utilize my experience.

Besides … you know my opinion about research and experts. Take ten of them; each will have his own opinion about what you should eat. What kind of science is that? Sadly, referring to science doesn't help you much if you don't do your own "research" as well. Experiment with your body to find what really works for you. Yes, you can use an expert's suggestions, but you need to take them with a grain of salt. Use your own judgment.

In the end it comes down to the trust you have in your source's reliability.

For nutrition and diet advice, I trust my friend, Matt Stone. He studies every piece of research on these topics he can find, in ridiculous detail. The guy knows more about the human body, its hormones, digestive system, etc., than many professors. He has dedicated the proverbial 10,000 hours to analyzing all available knowledge about health and fitness.

Matt Stone knows about the body.

As far as food goes, he's discovered that the the simplest and most impactful thing you can do is to eat non-processed foods.

I don't even understand most of the things he says about hormones and so on, but I easily grasped this: there is a direct correlation between the consumption of processed foods and the diseases which plague modern societies: cardiovascular system diseases responsible for strokes and heart attacks, diabetes, and cancers.

Scientists are trying to find the perfect diet to fight off those diseases by eliminating different kind of foods: sugar, fat, dairy, etc. They generally overlook, however, the fact that there are societies that are free from those diseases and yet still consume a lot of sugar, fats, dairy, and meat. But those societies consume these in their natural form, not processed.

A straightforward conclusion can be drawn here: you can eat a reasonable amount of dairy products or high-fat foods, which in themselves give nutrition, but not processed foods *containing* these nutritious elements. When we eat processed food, we're consuming the results of an artificial food production process, which is more difficult for our bodies to absorb.

Whatever the "label" on your present diet—Paleo, vegan, or something else—the best thing to energize your body is eating natural foods. Unfortunately, in most cases this means you need to cook your own food. Don't buy a burger in McDonalds; buy the piece of meat, a bread roll from the organic bakery, and veggies from the organic farm, and make the burger by yourself.

Your alternatives are to find places that serve meals made from natural ingredients or buy food from "eco" or "organic" shops. Usually these solutions are more expensive, both in money and time, as it takes a while to source and buy from out-of-the-way places.

But surely these alternatives are worth it. How much will a heart attack or cancer cost?

If you are new to finding the differences between natural and processed food, use this simple rule of thumb: was this food you are going to eat living somewhere a few days ago?

Think about the things you eat. Pizza doesn't grow on trees, apples do.

Another hack: ask yourself the process question. How much

work does it involve to make that food? For example, cottage cheese is definitely a processed food, but it takes just a few steps and a few ingredients to make it. It's white cheese and salt, nothing else.

To make a common white bread roll, you'll need fewer steps, and less additional chemical agents, than you'd need to make pizza. To make a roll you need just the processed flour. Pizza requires the same flour to make a base. But you'll need a bunch of other ingredients—cheese, sauce, and additions—to turn that bread base into dinner. Those additional items all contain the results of additional processes and chemicals. Your finished pizza is a chemical mixture without much nutritious value, which has all been "processed" out.

As the world's food production processes evolve, they remove more and more from the same basic food. The milk I add to coffee may be sterilized at a high temperature. I can choose also pasteurized milk, which employs lower temperatures in its production. Or I can choose to buy milk that is only mechanically filtered, directly from a farmer.

I agree with the natural food philosophy. As the statistical data about our civilization's diseases and processed food consumption indicate, the correlation between them is not accidental. Our ancestors lived shorter lives, but they died because of things most of us no longer face, such as mutilations, wounds, contagious infections, a poor quality water supply, and so on. We are dying now because our bodies—especially our hearts, livers, and kidneys — decline to function properly. Go back 50 years and compare stroke rates, cancer rates, heart attack rates, and diabetes rates to the current rates[ii]. "Surprisingly," fifty years ago, there was less technology involved in food production.

I have firsthand experience with natural foods. I have been eating at home my whole life. I very rarely feel the need or urge to eat out. And, surprise again, I'm healthy and always have been. My only chronic illness is an allergy and since I started paying attention to my health a couple years ago, it is much improved.

Of course, eating at home won't prevent you consuming processed foods. You can use processed ingredients (like white flour, for example) to cook your meals. However, if you pay attention to your cooking, it's much easier to eliminate processed food this way than by eating out. You always know—or should—what you put into the pot.

Here is another hack I recommend: cook your own version of unhealthy foods like cakes, pizzas, or burgers. No, do not buy prepared frozen products and heat them in the microwave! If you want to eat pizza, take flour, water, free range or barn eggs, and make a pie. Make sauce from the basic ingredients. Add meat from a known source, and some organic vegetables. Your pizza will be much healthier than anything you can get at a restaurant.

However, the healthfulness of one cake or pizza is just a side benefit. The biggest advantage of learning to cook everything from basic ingredients is that you'll quickly give up on those kinds of foods. It is an unbelievable amount of work to cook anything complex like pizza if you prepare all the bits yourself, especially if you are not used to doing it. The rule "I eat only what I prepared myself" is likely to turn you away from fancy foods fast.

Remember:

- The simplest and most impactful diet rule is: eat non-processed foods
- The simple rule of thumb to discern between natural and processed food is: was this food you are going to eat living somewhere a few days ago?

Action Items:

- Look your own meals (especially unhealthy foods)
- Learn how to read and understand product labels
- If you eat out or buy ingredients, pay attention to what you consume the same way you do when cooking on your own.

** FREE BONUS **

To download a single PDF sheet describing diet rules, visit:

www.ExpandBeyondYourself/diet

9. FASTING IS NOT FATAL

Decisions about how often and how much to eat are tough.

In the numerous and contradictory diet advice books, the recommended time and number of meals is as confusing as everything else in the health industry (what to eat, how to train, etc.). Some advocate eating a hefty breakfast, some just 30 g of protein first thing in the morning. Some advise to eat small meals frequently, others advise just a couple of large feasts. Some warn before eating in the evening, while their adversaries say it doesn't matter.

Do any of them really know anything?

As with everything else, you need to determine your *own* golden rule about what and when to eat. It needs to be something that is workable, which you can keep.

I have found merit in intermittent fasting.

In the Western world we are used to eating at least three meals a day. Breakfast is usually relatively early, after we awake or before work or school. We eat dinners late in the afternoon or early evening. We don't give our digestive systems time to rest and rejuvenate.

I believe fourteen hours is the minimal period of rest you should give your stomach. However, if you eat anything during the time between supper and breakfast, anything at all, you automatically shorten this break.

Every piece of food (well, the scientific rule of thumb says anything above 50 calories, so for example a couple of spoons of sugar) added on the top of your last meal, extends the time it takes your body to digest this additional fuel.

Your stomach needs rest as much as your brain or muscles. You can't solve complex problems for 20 hours a day. You can't lift weights 20 hours a day. You can't digest 20 hours a day. If you ate a steak at dinner, it could take as long as 8 hours to digest it. Give your stomach a break!

It's not strange that you feel out of energy every day if you spend a lot of energy on simply gaining energy from the huge amount of food you require your digestive system to process. Your gut is working overtime. It's only natural it's out of steam, and it will take even longer to digest food.

Stop overloading yourself. It's a vicious cycle. Give your body a rest, so it can burn up every scrap of nourishment you've put into it. Let it rest a few hours.

If you are one of the rare birds who eats the last meal around 6 p.m. and doesn't eat breakfast earlier than 8 a.m., feel free to skip the rest of this chapter. You're already providing the minimum 14-hour break for your hardworking stomach.

To preserve my energy in the morning, I don't eat till about 9 or 10 a.m. Then I consume only veggies and fruits. They are digested a lot faster than carbs or meat. When I eat my first meal about noon, my stomach is regenerated and ready for the challenge. However, I need energy during my working hours, so I don't eat excessively before 5 p.m. I provide my body just a few calories to burn up while I work.

Mainstream "wisdom" says that fasting is of religious origin, thus it's suspect. What do those fanatics know? They are harming their bodies, poor zealots.

I say, indeed! Fasting has a religious origin, thus it is trustworthy. Amazingly, despite conflicting beliefs on most issues, all main religions recommend the practice of fasting. It's clearly good both for the body and for the mind.

Only quite recently, scientists have been examining how fasting influences human metabolism and behavior. And many researchers confirm that intermittent fasting is beneficial. Really? Monks and priests knew this thousands of years ago. I don't want to sit on my hands for another century or two, until "conventional wisdom," or the FDA, agrees exactly how long the periods of fasting should be and when fasting is optimal.

I recommend you don't wait for anyone else to decide for you, either.

The two main arguments against fasting are based on prejudices rather than any solid facts. The first argument is that fasting is somehow philosophically "iffy," because religion has something to do with that. I don't accept that argument for a moment. The second argument tries to make the case that fasting will surely starve you. I'm not buying that one either.

Our tragic history has proved quite strongly that people can live without food for about a month. Moderate intermittent fasting won't kill you. Extreme fasting won't kill you. At the beginning of 2014, I fasted for 96 hours, ate a bowl of chicken soup, and fasted for 24 hours more. I survived. In the past week, I have fasted 135 hours out of 168. I survived.

From August to mid-October 2014, I ate only every other day and often I fasted 48 or even 72 hours in a row. At the end of this period, I looked like Angelina Jolie, but I survived. My fitness performance didn't degrade. In fact, I beat several personal records in that period reaching 66 dips, 43 pull-ups, and 45 chin-ups. My health was just fine. I didn't even have a headache.

I learned a lot about myself at that time. I could closely observe how my mind constantly whined for scraps of food. I practiced self-awareness and self-control.

We are talking about creating a successful body in this book, but intermittent fasting goes beyond that—it also provides you with a strong mind. When you fast, you can see how a scarcity of food affects you. You can observe firsthand how your brain tricks you into breaking your promises or into indulging yourself. A ton of self-help books and numerous "feel-good" messages might not convince you about the power of your subconscious, but just fast for a couple of days and you will experience this power personally.

The benefits of intermittent fasting include higher energy levels (on average), increased clarity and focus, easier weight control, and savings for your pocket. When you fast regularly, you kill two birds with one stone because when you eat less often, you also, naturally enough, often eat less. Fasting also wakes up your awareness about what you eat. My experience—and I'm not the only one who has observed this—is that when I started paying attention to the times of my meals, I also started paying more attention to what I consumed. It's just the normal feedback mechanism in your mind. When you focus on a subject, your internal filtering mechanism starts to pass up more information concerning it.

Fasting can be also a great mechanism for rapid weight loss. Thanks to my 120-hour fast, I lost pounds I had gained during Christmas. When I started my every-other-day fast, I weighed 144 lbs. When I finished it, I was 131 lbs. But it's not a weight-loss silver bullet. After Christmas in 2014, I was again 144 lbs. I definitely lost control of my sweet tooth this holiday. To maintain your weight for a long period of time, you need a sustainable lifestyle, not starving contests.

Maintaining an optimal weight involves more than just periods of abstaining from eating and periods of indulgence. It involves your mind. As long as you are in control of what goes into your mouth (or doesn't), everything is fine. If you lose control, you can finish on one side of the spectrum (anorexia) or the other (obesity). As with everything else (the most vivid example being money), intermittent fasting is a great tool if you control it, and a machine of destruction if it controls you.

I won't sell you on the "perfect" fasting plan. It's your life, your body and only you are allowed to experiment on yourself. I just invite you to perform some experiments. Try eating only 8 hours a day for a week. Abstain from food for 24 or 48 hours. Supervise your mood, energy levels, and performance. Research on the Internet what works for others. Some eat only one huge meal a day, others eat a few meals, but rigidly stick with the "eating for 8 hours only" rule, and others still fast 24 hours regularly every week.

While starting your experiments, aim to create a sustainable routine. Yes, I survived a one-time 120-hour fast, but I can assure you I am not able to sustain such a regime. The same goes with my two months of eating only every other day. For about 70 days it was an interesting experience, but later on it was beyond sensible.

What really works well for me is maintaining a 14-hour fast every day and coupling fasting with my religious beliefs; I don't eat on Fridays. It gives me motivation beyond mere physical results and really helps me to stick to this discipline. I encourage you to try to do the same with your fasting plan.

Go beyond the mundane and physical. Going hungry most of the time is not much fun. However, when it serves a higher purpose, like gaining self-control or improving your spiritual life, it's much easier to maintain.

Remember:

- Your stomach needs rest as much as your brain or muscles
- Intermittent fasting provides you with a strong mind
- Fasting can be a great mechanism for rapid weight loss, but it's not a silver bullet; beware the yo-yo effect.

Action Items:

- • Perform some fasting experiments: try eating only 8 hours a day for a week or abstain from food for 24 or 48 hours; supervise your mood, energy levels, and performance
- • Look for motivation beyond the physical; couple your fasting with a higher purpose.

** FREE BONUS **

To download a single PDF sheet describing my fasting strategy, visit:

www.ExpandBeyondYourself/fasting

10. VARIETY AND WEIGHT CONTROL

This is the part of the book dedicated to food, so it's time for some dietary advice. You had some glimpses about my nutritional beliefs in the previous chapters, but here I'll explain in detail what you should eat. No, not really.

The thing is, only nutcases (in this case, dietary fanatics) are convinced that this or that specific diet will make you free, errr … healthy. In my opinion, the *kind* of food you eat is not really that important. I don't think there is a perfect proportion of carbs, fats, proteins, fruits, and veggies.

There are people who thrive on a vegan diet. Others swear by the Paleo diet or have always eaten a Mediterranean diet, yet are doing well. A successful body is not achieved through eating specific kind of foods, but through becoming conscious about what is good for you and knowingly sticking to that.

I think that the moderation rule works very well in this regard. That's my approach to eating. All kinds of foods have a place in my diet: vegetables, fruits, proteins, fats, carbs … well, sugar has no place in it, but the stuff always finds a way to sneak into my day; I'm a lifelong sweets addict. To temper my cravings, I allow myself to eat a natural honey. As I explained in Chapter 8, I try to eat more natural foods than processed ones, and that's my only firm "food rule."

While pursuing the weight-loss quest described in my book *The Fitness Expert Next Door* (you can grab it for free on Amazon and Smashwords), I found veggies and fruits very helpful for keeping my weight under control. These are low-calorie foods and are great for occupying my mind and stomach as replacements for the high-calorie, less-healthy foods I crave.

This variety is really what allows me to maintain my weight. Since March 2013, I've kept my weight in the 136–144 lbs. range (except during my flirt with extended fasting, that is). When I'm bored with one kind of food, I try another one. When I observe that my sweets cravings are affecting my sanity, I allow myself a donut or two (or two pounds of cake).

Your body and mind just do not seem to retain valuable lessons from the past and need to be reminded from time to time. It's like alcohol and a hangover. Right after a big party, when you went too far, your lesson is reinforced, and you're revolted by even the thought of alcohol. But a month or two later, you'll have "temporary amnesia," and you'll convince yourself that this time it won't be so bad … but you'll again regret your actions afterward.

I *know* that sweets disrupt my hormonal equilibrium. I *know* that it's the fastest way to grow my spare-tire belly. But I've also discovered that I can't reasonably argue with my body. It has to experience the drawbacks of certain choices now and then before it will resubmit to my arguments. It's like a little child: *"But dad, this time we surely won't gain weight. Let's try indulgence once again; it feels sooooo good."*

I've found out that my overall energy expenditure is less if I allow occasional lessons that remind my inner child of nature's unchanging laws (eating that food = gaining weight, fool). It takes a *lot* of willpower to keep an iron grip on your diet, and sometimes the energy is better spent elsewhere.

Once again, it's a tricky thing, as with fasting. You must watch yourself so you don't give up control to your inner child too often. But in the case of weight, it's quite easy to be checked. You know, there is a device called a scale. Use it regularly (I weigh myself once a week) and you will get the necessary reality check.

I've been assuming you already know why you should keep an optimal weight. But one should never assume. So here is the sermon:

I was overweight and I am not anymore. Life is much better for me today. The only advantage I can find for being okay with being overweight is that you don't have to think about your diet at all. If you don't have to think about it, this saves considerable time that the weight-conscious lot spend "unnecessarily" on exercise, cooking healthy meals, buying natural foods, and considering if they've had enough already or can afford a few bites more.

But disadvantages override this timesaver by a long shot.

When overweight, I had less energy because my stomach was

46

digesting something almost all the time. I slept more to regain my energy. When it came to the simplest physical activities, like running to the bus station in the morning, I was exhausted. But being overweight affected far more than just my energy. Succumbing to my cravings diminished my willpower and self-control. I was content with my life as soon as I put something sweet in my mouth. I firmly believe it's not an accident that my mindset transformation took place about half a year after I started my fight to lose weight. I trained my "willpower muscle" and my energy level improved, so I was able to look for more in my life than just going through the next day.

And that "advantage" you get when you don't worry about being overweight? From what I see, it's an illusion. Overweight people lose more time down the road waiting in queues for doctors (or waiting for the next bus, because they didn't run fast enough to catch the previous one!).

I can't tell you why being underweight sucks because I never have been (you must ask Angelina Jolie about this). Even at 130 lbs., I was still in my optimal BMI range. But I'm sure it sucks as much as being overweight. Moderation is the key to a successful body, and eating is the key to optimal body weight. If your body weight is outside the optimal Body Mass Index boundaries, I seriously encourage you to take some steps to change it. The majority of modern society has a problem with an excessive mass, and getting to your optimal weight means shedding some fat.

Yes, there are successful, overweight people out there. It's not that this is an impassable obstacle to success in many fields, although carrying excess weight will make some tasks *very* difficult. Overweight people have chosen the harder path. Apart from the usual struggles that happen when one tries to achieve something massive in life, they also have to struggle with their health and energy levels.

Optimal body weight equates with optimal energy level.

Here are three quick tips that will help with "downgrading" your body: keep a food journal, eat smaller portions, and switch from high-calorie foods (cakes and burgers) to low-calorie foods (carrots and apples).

To summarize this chapter, I recommend a diet called "your diet." It is the one that allows you to keep an optimal body weight and energy level, not the one your friend (or even your doctor) recommends. "Your diet" should be one you can sustain (think ten years or more).

Remember:

- There is no such a thing as a perfect diet
- Staying overweight makes everything harder
- Optimal body weight equates with optimal energy level
- Your diet should be sustainable for at least ten years.

Action Items:

- • Use a device called a scale to get the necessary reality check
- • Get to know your BMI and try to stay in the normal-weight range.

** FREE BONUS **

To download a single PDF sheet describing my weight maintenance strategy, visit:

www.ExpandBeyondYourself/weight

11. DRINKING PROBLEM

No, not alcohol drinking. Alcohol is highly calorific and, when used in excess, causes the death of gray cells in your brain, which is pretty much irreparable. But this chapter is not a sermon about what you should not drink. (Okay, I'll make an exception for soda. That stuff contains excessive calories, is addictive, and there is no high after it. I can see no reason anyone should drink soda.)

I want to highlight the importance of water.

About 90 percent of your body is water. It is important to drink water. As a society, we are generally dehydrated. This changed a bit with the fashion for drinking bottled water, but that fad is popular mainly among health fanatics.

An ordinary man has generally too many worries to pay much attention to drinking water. No one he knows has died from thirst, so what's this fuss about? Well, it's about health. If you frequently don't drink enough water, it undermines your health. If you constantly keep the right water balance, you are okay. It's as simple as that.

But how much is the golden measure? It's for you to determine. I imagine that a guy who is seven feet tall and weighs 240 pounds needs a bit more water than a 5'5" peanut like me. The rule of thumb is 2 liters a day (about 68 oz.). But if you live in the tropics, or if you work physically 8 hours a day, you need to drink more, of course.

Unlike with food, it is quite important when you drink. You should drink continually: A glass of water just after you wake, a glass of water before you go to work, a glass of water after dinner, and a glass of water before you go to bed. You should be continually replenishing your body with a steady stream of fluids.

I'm quite fond of drinking a glass of water first thing in the morning. I introduced this habit last year and don't regret it at all. The only tangible effect I can pinpoint is a lack of headaches. They'd been my nightmare since childhood. When I was a teenager, I had regular migraines. About the age of sixteen they diminished, but I inevitably still suffered a hefty headache a few times a year.

However, during the last eighteen months, I've had only one serious headache. The habit of drinking a glass of water just after sleep was relatively easy to develop. My body got used to the fact that a glass of water would be provided within the first ten minutes after waking up and it appropriately regulated its mechanisms. Nowadays, I'm always thirsty after sleep, whereas a couple of years ago I couldn't ingest anything for up to three hours after I woke.

Why should you drink water and not coffee or tea?

The main reason for a *water* intake is to replenish the water in your body. A secondary but still significant reason is that drinking water tops up your body's microelements like sodium, magnesium, calcium, and potassium, if these are present. Other beverages tend to leach those elements from your body instead of providing them. Unfortunately, plain water with a low microelement content does the same.

That's the reason, if you're not drinking tap water, you should take notice of how many minerals are in the bottle. If the water contains less than 250 ppm of dissolved salts, then the tap water at your house is probably healthier. Frankly, finding bottled water that has a composition of minerals that justifies the exaggerated price is almost impossible.

Can an excess of water be harmful to your body? Yes, an excess of *anything* is usually harmful, and so it is with water. Drink two or three liters, but not five or ten. If you pump excessive fluid into yourself, you don't give your body time to assimilate those minerals. The water just comes through you, and your kidneys and bowel have to work overtime.

Remember:

- Drinking water is healthy
- On average, we drink too little water
- Drinking other beverages is less healthy
- Bottled water is not significantly better than tap water
- Drinking too much could be as negative as drinking too little.

Action Items:

- Drink water ;)

** FREE BONUS **

To download a single PDF sheet describing my hydration strategy, visit:

www.ExpandBeyondYourself/hydration

12. FITNESS SHORTCUT: HIGH-INTENSITY INTERVAL TRAINING

HIIT is an acronym that means High-Intensity Interval Training. It is "an enhanced form of interval training, an exercise strategy alternating periods of short intense anaerobic exercise with less-intense recovery periods.[iii]" As with everything else, specialists and enthusiasts can't agree how this definition should translate into a specific workout regime.

I don't argue idly with theoreticians or fanatics. I just train. My favorite way of doing workouts restricts intense exercise periods to just a single series of exercise. I make sure that it is hellishly intensive. Not just "high," but rather "orbital."

To give you a comparison, there is a specific HIIT workout protocol called a Tabata Protocol. It's very specific because it's based directly on the research published in 1996 by a professor at the Faculty of Sport and Health Science at Ritsumeikan University in Japan. The original research of Dr. Izumi Tabata indicated that his protocol offers more performance benefits in less time (than other exercise regimes), because it improved both the anaerobic energy system (i.e., the system responsible for short, high-intensity exercise, such as sprints) and the aerobic energy system (i.e., the system used for endurance exercise, such as long, slow running).

Tabata Protocol formula is very simple: 20 seconds of a very high-intensity exercise (like a sprint) followed by breaks of 10 seconds; the cycle is repeated eight times.

Additional studies confirmed Tabata's findings, and that's no surprise to me, nor is the reality that some scientists have come to the conclusion that HIIT may be downright deadly. Whoa! Don't expect science to explain your particular life, unless you are the object of a particular study. Learn, try, and make your own deductions.

My experience brought me to the same conclusions Dr. Tabata reached. HIIT training is the best bang for my buck or, rather, for my time. I need literally 3 minutes to fail doing pull-ups or a harder push-up variant. Trust me; after 45 chin-ups or 60 diamond push-ups or legs-elevated push-ups, you feel as exhausted as after 4 minutes of Tabata's workout. I don't need equipment or a gym to do my HIIT workout. I can do it anywhere. Very often I do it in the bathroom at the office.

The only restriction for this kind of training is that you need to already be in relatively good shape. If your blood circulation system isn't flawless, you would be better to start slow and go easy on yourself initially. However, when I was ten pounds overweight, I was still able to train that way, so it is not too limiting. You can do it!

An exercise regime alone isn't a good weight-loss strategy. I lost some pounds and inches, but mainly through changing my diet. I've been doing push-ups very intensively each morning for several years, but during that time I still put on pounds, to the point where I was overweight. Exercises alone won't overcome the effect of a sweet tooth (or any other eating vice).

Exercise is not my friend. I don't like extended physical effort. I don't like running. The longest run I've undertaken in my life (until quite recently) was one kilometer during PE while still in primary school. I was twelve then and still shudder at the memory of it.

The only extended exercise I somewhat like is swimming. I can swim for half an hour without a single break. Did I mention that I am a white-collar worker and spend eight hours a day behind a desk and four more commuting every day? My endurance and overall performance in any physical activity should suck, considering I train just about ten minutes a day, shouldn't it?

But during those ten minutes, I train with HIIT, which even in short periods like that will develop endurance.

A couple of months ago, when I left the office, I decided on a whim to run to the train station, which is a mile and a half from the office. I had my backpack with laptop (weight about eight pounds) and my winter coat. I started, I ran, and I made the whole distance without a single break. My time wasn't groundbreaking (it took me ten minutes) but the astounding fact—to me—is that I was able to do that at all!

Endurance is part of the benefit of HIIT; the other part is performance. With my extremely limited time investment, I was able to go from fourteen chin-ups about three and a half years ago to 46 now. When I restarted my push-ups habit in 2005 or 2006, I was doing fewer than 50 normal push-ups. Within a few years I could do more than 100 regularly, but it takes quite a lot of time to do 100 push-ups. I switched to harder and shorter push-up variants: legs-elevated, diamonds, wide-grip, narrow-grip, and knuckles. Then I invited my kids to sit on my back. That worked quite well until I started to wake up long before they did, and had to exercise without my "back weight."

Last month I decided to test how many normal push-ups I could do. I decided to sacrifice five to ten minutes for this test. I managed 147.

All of this is a nice self-confidence boost. I'm quite proud of my performance. But the most important result of my daily ultra-short trainings is not that I can do lots of push-ups. Rather, it is that I have more energy than my peers, and I maintain this high-energy balance without investing much time or effort and without needing a fancy diet. Four minutes a day is the minimum I need to maintain my energy level. My workmates run marathons and attend the gym or the swimming pool regularly to stay in shape. Nonetheless, the time commitment eats their schedules alive. I get the same or better results with almost no time commitment.

HIIT training is also great for your mind. It helps you develop a winner's attitude. When you train to the point of failure each day, you'll receive an understanding about the value of giving your best.

If you force your muscles each morning to produce everything you have, you are more likely to force your mind to do what you want to do. HIIT my way builds ability to focus, plus it builds self-control and willpower. See? It's just one simple activity, but it has so many advantages that it's a sin not to practice it or replace less effective methods with it.

Remember:

- HIIT improves both endurance and performance
- It gives the best benefit for your time investment
- HIIT helps you develop a winner's attitude.

Action Items:

- Try doing the Tabata Protocol; modify it to your needs (e.g., pull-ups series instead of sprint)
- Pick your favorite body-weight exercises (push-ups, pull-ups, burpees, etc.) and do one series of them to the point of failure every day.

** FREE BONUS **

To download a single PDF sheet describing my HIIT workout, visit:

www.ExpandBeyondYourself/hiit

13. STEADY STATE CARDIO

Let's discuss cardio, which is supposed to train your endurance.

In my experience, it's a waste of time. I can train my endurance just as well with HIIT.

The only advantage I see with cardio is the chance for socializing. You can run around your neighborhood and get to know your neighbors. Or you can go to the gym with your friends or business partners. Then you kill two birds with one stone: get fit and be with people.

I limit my cardio to doing a Weider series (aerobic exercises that flatten the stomach). I used to do it for about fifteen minutes in the morning every day; now I do it a few times a week. Anyway, during this exercise I listen to podcasts and audio programs. It's not the best way to learn something, but it's a great way to get ideas and "be" with people with attitudes and mindsets that are scarce in my local social environment. So when you properly use "cardio time," it's far from being a total waste.

Besides, some people just need other people to cheer them on, or they won't move their ass, no matter what. I'm an introvert. I would happily spend 22 hours a day alone. But some people (and this fact puzzles me to no end) actually like to be among other people. If they don't go to the gym and feel they are in a social environment where it's "cool" to exercise, there is no power in the universe that will force them into physical activity.

Others are just morbidly bored with "mere" training, and so can't stick to a routine. They might persevere for a week or two if a flash of determination hits, but soon boredom takes any initiative away. If that is you, then definitely train using cardio exercises. Any movement is better than no movement.

Another reason people love cardio is simple addiction. During extended physical effort (after about fifteen minutes) your body produces endorphins, the natural "happy" drug. This natural drug is as addictive as some chemical substances produced in laboratories and factories. If you can transform a grueling exercise—running—into a happy experience, my hearty congratulations. Keep at it! Happiness is sometimes so hard to achieve. (Of course, I could provide you with at least five easier and faster ways to be happy, just off of the top of my head, but let's not fix what's not broken.)

I've mentioned that breaking my personal records boosts my self-esteem. Cardio exercises may be as good an area for breaking records as pull-ups. When I ran my mile and a half to the train or swam 60 pool lengths for the first time, I was stoked in the same way. You can always put up some challenge and do your exercise longer or faster and take pride from your accomplishment. Breaking your own records is the best source of motivation and self-confidence because you aren't competing with anyone else. You are winning over yourself. The you from yesterday is the only person in the race. In short, it's an internal rather than external frame of reference, so it is much less likely to frustrate you.

There is research that "proves" cardio exercises are harmful. On reflection, I don't think cardio is intrinsically evil or wrong. The Maasai people of the African plains run long distances, often. Clearly, their culture has survived for centuries and their "cardio" hasn't killed them all off, indicating that it wasn't so harmful after all.

I'm sure there is a "best" way to do cardio, so as to draw the most benefit from it. I just don't know what that is, and I'm not too bothered, as I'm getting great results from HIIT.

Therefore, I'm recommending the use of cardio for fitness only to encourage action over inaction. If your social conditioning or personal preferences are on the side of cardio, go for it. I think you are better off spending hours on a treadmill than on the couch.

Remember:

- Cardio is supposed to improve your endurance
- It's a great way to get some exercise and socialize (or learn) at the same time.

** FREE BONUS **

To download a single PDF sheet describing my cardio workout, visit:

www.ExpandBeyondYourself/cardio

14. I LIKE TO MOVE IT, MOVE IT

Having an established workout routine is fine and good. I personally know some individuals that just hate the very thought of working out. They are all but allergic to the word (most of them suffer from Failed New Year's Resolution Syndrome). Does it mean they are doomed to be fat and weak? Not at all.

To have a successful body you don't need to be a weight lifting champion, or even as crazy about pull-ups as I am. All you need is to move regularly. If you hate the idea of exercise, try the playful approach. Play some sport. One of my card-game buddies is very overweight. When you carry a few dozen needless fat pounds everywhere you go, you are constantly tired. The very thought of exercise is off-putting.

My buddy doesn't exercise. But he plays. Every week he plays volleyball with a group of friends for a couple of hours. He is still overweight. With all the soda he drinks, it's unavoidable. (He works for the soda factory, poor fellow.) But he at least moves his ass on a regular basis.

This volleyball my friend plays is not a programmed fitness scheme he's devised; he just plays with his friends and gets exercise doing it. By no means will this routine make him a fitness model, but even a small amount of physical activity is better than nothing. If he wasn't playing volleyball, he would be in a much worse state. I shudder to contemplate it.

Does the word *exercise* trigger an alarm in your head? Try some sport instead. You should look for a sport that is both enjoyable and accessible for you so you will be able to keep at it and perform it regularly. It's no good if you love ice hockey but live in Florida and can play ice hockey only when you visit your grandpa in Canada once a year. A tennis court next door is no use if you can't or don't like to play tennis. Both conditions must be met so you can use your chosen sport for building a successful body. If you can't cope with regular exercises, you must replace them with some other regular activity.

The more often you can play your favorite sport, the better.

Action creates momentum, and you'll move more and reap the benefits of it faster by keeping the momentum going.

In case you wondered, neither poker nor chess count as exercise.

I see. You shudder at the thought of a workout in your schedule, and you just don't enjoy any sport. Your case is hopeless, then. Just kidding.

Nonetheless, you'll seriously limit your chances for developing a successful body if you can't or won't do any form of planned consistent movement. It's really hard to create and preserve a high level of energy by sitting on the couch. You will need to find more opportunities to move about.

Try to develop new habits that will help you do that in everyday life situations. I have a sedentary job, so besides my HIIT workouts, I've developed a few such habits to enhance my physiology. For example, my house has an upper level where we have our bedrooms. My home office is on the ground floor. I need to run up seventeen steps each time I want anything from the other level. I don't just go up or down the stairs. I run every time. It's a mini workout, especially when I am cooking a dinner in the kitchen downstairs and simultaneously helping my daughter with homework upstairs.

Away from home, I try to run stairs every time I encounter them. My work is on the third floor of a building, so I have stairs there to run up every day. As a rule I don't use an elevator unless I'm going up farther than the tenth floor. I can also choose to run to my bus. Between the office I work in and the bus stop, it is about 500 yards. I don't return home by bus every day, but every time I take this route, I run this distance instead of walking it.

Such small habits are relatively easy to develop. These can be melded into your everyday life so you get ongoing benefit. It's possible you face stairs, elevators, and a road to work every single day. Plan to use these "obstacles" as opportunities! Once you develop a stepping-up-the-game habit, you will likely stick with it for the rest of your life. And you will enjoy the benefits for the rest of your life.

After some time, you will stop consciously thinking about whether to avoid an elevator, or if you should run up the stairs. When behavior turns habitual, you no longer think about it; your actions are ingrained. When you encounter stairs, you'll start to run. Or you'll go up a few first steps walking, and catch yourself doing it. That's what your subconscious does; it prompts you when there's something "not normal" in a situation.

Won't it be great when that happens with your exercise habits? The cues that trigger habits are hooked so deep inside you, that when you don't react to one, you'll automatically feel uneasy, because you'll feel that something is wrong:

"Oh, I'm walking instead of running."

Of course, the opportunity to move a bit more or faster in your life isn't restricted to just the stairs you come across. Analyze your day. You'll surely find multiple opportunities for moving more. When you go to the mall, leave a car at the parking place farthest from the entrance. Or stop using shopping carts and carry your shopping bags. If your commute to work is relatively short, try cycling instead of driving.

Another great chance to move more is reserved for parents only. Well, you can always make friends with people with kids, if you don't have your own.

Playing with kids can be more exhausting than moderate workouts. Those little monsters have infinite reservoirs of energy. Playing tag or any team game like baseball or basketball with kids can wear you out in no time. It's fun and your body will be forced to move like a hamster spinning its wheel. You won't have time to think about repetitions or weights when you play with kids; you just play, and you'll get fit along the way.

As you know now, I'm a firm believer in consistency. I encourage you to develop some playing rituals with your kids. Play with them every Sunday; a basketball match, perhaps. Or play tag for ten minutes every day after you return from work. This activity is not just good for your body; it will bond you together. I employed my kids to help with my push-ups, and they still try to climb on top when they see me doing them, even my fourteen-year-old, who is bigger and heavier than me!

Physical activities with your kids are much more engaging than mundane workouts at the gym. Nonetheless, one can be as exhausting as the other. If every other scheme for moving more has failed, use this one. The effects are guaranteed.

Remember:

- Consistency is the key
- You don't have to exercise; you have to move regularly.

Action Items:

- Try playing sports, smuggling physical activity into everyday life, or playing with your kids on a regular schedule

- Take a pen and a sheet of paper and brainstorm at least five everyday activities you can use to move more; implement one ASAP.

** FREE BONUS **

To download a single PDF sheet describing how I maintain my routine, visit:

www.ExpandBeyondYourself/consistency

15. CAN YOU HAVE A SUCCESSFUL BODY?

Of course you can. You are a human being; your body is one of the important elements of your persona and you can modify it. It's not about lifting tons of dumbbells or having a six-pack on your belly. It's about having enough energy every day to sustain you in your quest for a better life.

It's not a question of time or willpower. You always have 24 hours a day. It's you who decide how you will use them. Your health, as represented by the state of your body, is the most basic element of who you are. If you don't find time to take care of it, how can you find time for activities you have far less power over like, let's say, publishing a book?

Publishing books is a complex activity involving a lot of other people and work. And it takes time to interact with those people and a dedication to that work. Here is the secret about cooperating with other people: you can't govern them like you can govern the parts of your body. Forcing yourself to do 100 push-ups is childishly easy in comparison to trying to force a cover designer to provide what you want, when you want it.

The truth is that you always find time for the things you want to do. Do you want a successful body? Then you will find the time to prepare your own meals or to go to the gym regularly. Then you will figure out how to accommodate your schedule and actually sleep seven hours a day. But if this desire doesn't come from within you, you will find only excuses. You will find time and opportunities in your life to watch TV for hours or to indulge yourself with fast food.

Will you succeed?

Let us define failure. The only way to fail is to stop trying. A strong body with good health is a necessary prerequisite to real success. Having one frees additional energy for you, so you can have a more fulfilled life. If you are exhausted after work, it's hard to find energy to play with your kids or do homework with them. It's hard to be a charming guy who will date your wife and win her heart once again.

I believe a healthy body is a prerequisite for just about everything.

You can't give up on your health.

Keep trying. Be persistent and do something every day to improve it. Once you achieve a satisfying level of energy, be mindful and don't slip into your old ways. While developing new ways to enhance your well-being, remember that they have to be sustainable. Your body will be with you to the very end. There is no use in figuring out how to lose 30 pounds of fat in three months, if in the next three months after that you gain back 33 pounds.

High energy is absolutely crucial to your personal success. The hardest work in the world is to keep the right mindset, to keep thinking and focusing on your principal goal. Exercising is easy. Writing is easy. Doing business is easy. Solving problems is easy. But keeping your mind absorbed on those things long enough for momentum to kick in, consumes unbelievable amounts of energy.

If your body cannot be your support system because it is more of a liability than an asset, then everything is twice as hard. It's of course possible to be disabled or chronically sick and succeed. It's just so fricking hard. Do yourself a favor and take care of your health, so the rest of your life can be put together more easily.

That's my message to you: if you are not disabled, work on making your body successful. It's very unlikely that you will achieve anything meaningful with a weak ruin of a body. Well, unless you want to invent and sell a "Success for low-energy folks" program.

Improve your sleeping, eating, and exercising habits slightly, keep those new routines for at least 30 days, and you will notice a positive difference. This is actually as close to an instant feedback system as you'll ever get.

Take writing, in contrast. I wrote my first booklet, which was under 10,000 words, within 45 days. During that time, I had almost zero feedback about my work. I shared it with my friends, but their opinion was a bit biased (putting it mildly). It was an additional two weeks before it was proofread, formatted, and uploaded on Amazon.

Then I waited another month to get meaningful results. Can you imagine how that was messing with my mind?

All that time I had to persevere, with only hope and faith that my effort would be justified in the end. And it was. I've sold more than a thousand copies of that book, and given away a few thousand more during free promotions. But it was very hard to be convinced that success was coming when I had sold just 130 copies of it within the first seven months.

It's not so hard with your body.

We are so effective in harming our bodies, that when we stop doing it, improvements are visible immediately. If you sleep six hours a day, try to sleep seven and a half hours for just one week. In just one week you will feel the difference. If you are dehydrated, start drinking more water. You will be amazed how fast your headaches will be gone. If you are living on a fast food diet, switch to whole foods for a couple of weeks. You'll feel like you flipped a switch in your body from "minimal energy" to "high energy."

Unfortunately, exercising doesn't give such clear, immediate results. Try to work out intensively for a week and you will feel sore and sorry. But the effect of exercise is cumulative too. You just need to go through the initial painful period to reap the benefits.

The instant feedback loop about your efforts is great, especially at the beginning. Our internal constitution, at a superficial level, is wired for instant feedback. I guess our ancestors had to learn to throw straight or die of hunger. Whatever the reasons, our subconscious mind doesn't really grasp the concept of time. It expects results *now*. When they don't come immediately, it resists spending any further energy on activities that seem to bring no benefits. Thus, immediate results help you to stay motivated by providing more energy for further effort.

However, there is also a danger involved with quick results: that you will notice these positive results and stop your exertions. Or you'll think "just one cake won't matter," since things are going so well. All in all, you may reason, why slog more, as it's obviously pretty simple to get what you want?

You must keep in mind that at the beginning (if you want long-term results), you shouldn't pursue results *per se*, but rather consistency. You don't just want results today; you want a system that brings results for the rest of your life.

Whenever you undertake some extreme measure (like a three-day fast), "explain" to your subconscious that it's just temporary. Agree with yourself about your purpose: you're doing it to cleanse or to shed some fat. Then you will be less likely to have to fight with yourself over it.

While in pursuit of your successful body, I strongly encourage you to make small changes in what may be a mundane series of day-to-day activities, rather than invent any complex schemes. A small change in diet (carrots replacing cookies), going to bed a bit earlier, introducing ten minutes of exercises into your mornings, and so on; all these are easy to implement and bring tangible, quick results.

For permanent change, you need sustainable disciplines that will keep you going far into the future. The best changes are the ones you can stick with to your last day on this planet.

Remember:

- Yes, you can
- High energy is absolutely crucial to your personal success
- At the beginning you shouldn't pursue results per se, but rather consistency.

Action Items:

- Be persistent and do something every day to improve your health
- Implement small changes one by one
- Answer right now: which discipline will you implement first?

16. SUCCESS THROUGH YOUR BODY

The foremost advantage you'll get with a successful body is more energy. If your health is vibrant, you'll be able to do so much more—with your body, with your mind, and with your time. Doors will open to new opportunities. You'll have free energy to dream again, to think with clarity, to work with a diligent focus. You'll find yourself happier, and your happiness will rub off on those around you. When you have more energy, you'll be freer to lighten the burden on your spouse by taking more responsibilities on your shoulders. The same can happen in your workplace. You will have more strength to play with your children.

The list of possible benefits is almost endless.

It's not a theory. We admire people who can give their best in any possible realm. John Lee Dumas works about sixteen hours every Monday to record seven episodes of his podcast. Top sportsmen are admired for how far they can push their bodies. It's often extraordinary how they can keep up a fast pace on the field, and at the same time think about overall strategy and the tactics for the next few moves.

I know and admire stay-at-home mothers who have five and more kids. A gal I know has eight, and she got a master's degree in the middle of that turmoil.

I wasn't always a productivity machine, cranking out a thousand words a day with machine-like regularity, while working a full-time job and taking care of my family of five. There was an exact correlation between taking better care of my body and releasing creative juices and endurance to keep going. Most folks who know me consider me at least a bit crazy. For the last couple of years, I worked almost every single day and I worked at least ten hours each day. I cease work only for the holy days of my religion; luckily, every Sunday counts as such.

In the spring of 2012 I decided to do something about my bulging gut. I managed to get rid of about eight pounds by eliminating most sweets from my diet. And then I read *The Slight Edge*. My energy level had increased enough to make me curious about life outside my small cozy world and to ponder some uncomfortable thoughts about my future. That led me to improving my diet and exercise regime even further, releasing even more energy.

Cultivating your health is like digging a well in a desert. At the beginning, it seems to be a fruitless slog. But once the spring is revealed, the water may be used in so many applications that you don't really know how to maximize it. It creates abundance. It supplies your mind and soul with creative ideas and sufficient positive feeling that you're motivated to stretch and try them out.

The increased energy is just the first fruit of a successful body. The next one is the realization that you actually have power over your life. This feedback loop I talked about in the previous chapter opens your eyes to the fact that *you* have power over your mind, that your mind dictates your actions, and that your actions shape who you are and shape the world around you.

This feedback loop is as close to instant as you can get. The majority of people who decide to lose weight and dedicate some effort to that goal can observe the result of their efforts on the scale within a couple of weeks. That's fast! Try starting a new business and getting results in that time frame. Decide to become a professional sportsman and start training for tennis or basketball. Your skills after two weeks will still be laughable. You'll need to slog for a long period of time, usually without any tangible confirmation that your efforts will take you where you want to be, before you can attain such lofty goals.

You need a successful mindset to do that. And working on, and with, your body will develop such a mindset for you. Yes, realize that you can.

Another benefit of developing a successful body is increased self-esteem. Being fit among a population of overweight individuals (almost 70 percent of Americans are overweight) makes you stand out. You feel better about yourself. You feel more in control. Your belief in your abilities grows. Your health related accomplishments make you proud of yourself. You feel empowered. You change your self-talk; after all, you are the person who talks to you the most in the whole world.

Being only slightly overweight, I was more or less immune to my wife's and friends' teasing. My life was good overall, and my weight wasn't a self-esteem issue for me. But it became an issue when I managed to lose some weight. I achieved success. I now revel in the self-esteem my fitness gives me. It has been rising, too. It jumps a bit more each time I beat another personal fitness record. I have beaten a lot of them within the last two years, over 80 since I started my online progress journal.

More energy, higher self-esteem, and increased awareness about what you are able to do with your life are only a beginning. From those foundations, your life transformation will start. You'll be able to think with conviction about pursuing success, however you define it.

A successful body gives you strength for the marathon called life. It will supply whatever energy you need, day by day, year after year. Once you realize the benefits you're getting, taking proper care of your body will quickly become an obsession. You'll be glued to your healthy disciplines. You'll maintain your habits with para-religious zeal. You will find yourself with unstoppable momentum, able to go after whatever dreams you have. You'll be ready for every challenge life will bring you. You'll be ready for success.

That's your destiny. Now go and start developing a successful body.

It's within your reach.

<<<< The End >>>>

CONNECT WITH MICHAL

Thanks for reading all the way to the end. If you made it this far, you must have liked it! I really appreciate having people all over the world take interest in the thoughts, ideas, research, and words that I share in my books. I appreciate it so much that I invite you to visit www.ExpandBeyondYourself.com, where you can register to receive all of my future releases absolutely free.

Read a manifesto on my blog and if it clicks with you, there is a sign-up form at the bottom of the page, so we can stay connected.

Once again, that's

www.ExpandBeyondYourself.com

More Books by Michal Stawicki

You can find more books by Michal at:

www.ExpandBeyondYourself.com/about/my-books/

A Small Favor

I want to ask a favor of you. If you have found value in this book, please take a moment and share your opinion with the world. Just let me know what you learned and how it affected you in a positive way. Your reviews help me to positively change the lives of others. Thank you!

About the Author

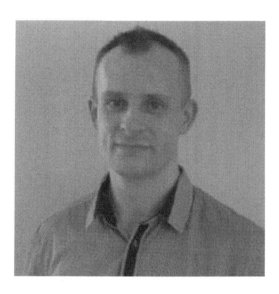

I'm Michal Stawicki and I live in Poland, Europe. I've been married for over fifteen years and am the father of two boys and one girl. I work full time in the IT industry, and recently, I've become an author. My passions are transparency, integrity, and progress.

In August 2012, I read a book called *The Slight Edge* by Jeff Olson. It took me a whole month to start implementing ideas from this book. That led me to reading numerous other books on personal development, some effective, some not so much. I took a look at myself and decided this was one person who could surely use some development.

In November of 2012, I created my personal mission statement; I consider it the real starting point of my progress. Over several months' time, I applied numerous self-help concepts and started building inspiring results: I lost some weight, greatly increased my savings, built new skills, and got rid of bad habits while developing better ones.

I'm very pragmatic, a down-to-earth person. I favor utilitarian, bottom-line results over pure artistry. Despite the ridiculous language, however, I found there is value in the "hokey-pokey visualization" stuff and I now see it as my mission to share what I have learned.

My books are not abstract. I avoid going mystical as much as possible. I don't believe that pure theory is what we need in order to change our lives; the Internet age has proven this quite clearly. What you will find in my books are:

- Detailed techniques and methods describing how you can improve your skills and drive results in specific areas of your life

- Real life examples

- Personal stories

So, whether you are completely new to personal development or have been crazy about the Law of Attraction for years, if you are looking for concrete strategies, you will find them in my books. My writing shows that I am a relatable, ordinary guy and not some ivory tower guru.

Endnotes:

[i]

http://www.viktorfrankl.org/e/lifeandwork.html

[ii] Mortality rates are slowly declining, but incidence rates are steadily climbing.

http://circ.ahajournals.org/content/125/1/e2/F12.expansion.html

http://onlinelibrary.wiley.com/doi/10.3322/caac.20073/pdf

[iii] Says Wikipedia:
http://en.wikipedia.org/wiki/High-intensity_interval_training

42357490R00048

Made in the USA
San Bernardino, CA
02 December 2016